EVERYTHING ABOUT

CARB CYCLING

DIET

Complete Nutritional Cookbook, Foods, Meal Plan, Recipes And A Guide To Helping You Lose Weight, Improve Sporting Performance, And Increase Insulin Sensitivity

DR. ALVIN BRANTLEY

Disclaimer

The information provided in this book is intended for general informational purposes only. It is not a substitute for professional medical advice, diagnosis, or treatment.

You should not use the information in this book for diagnosing or treating a health problem or disease by self decision. Always seek the advice of your physician or other qualified health provider with any questions you may have regarding a medical condition.

The author and publisher of this book make no representations or warranties with respect to the accuracy, applicability, fitness, or completeness of the contents of this book. The information contained in this book is based on the author's research and experience, and it is shared with the understanding that the author is not engaged in rendering medical, health, or any other kind of professional advice for you by this book.

The author does not endorse or promote any specific products, brands, or companies related to the contents provided in this book.

Any mention of products or services in this book is for informational purposes only and does not constitute an endorsement.

The author has not entered into any affiliate marketing agreements and has not signed any endorsement deals with individuals, organizations, or companies.

Readers are encouraged to consult with their healthcare providers before making any dietary or lifestyle chaSnges based on the information provided in this book. The author and publisher disclaim any liability for the decisions made by readers based on the information in this book.

Contents

Introduction

One essential macronutrient that the body uses as its main source of energy is carbohydrates. Carbohydrates are made up of sugars, fibers, and starches. During digestion, they are broken down into glucose, which is used as fuel for several body processes. For people who are thinking about using a carb cycling technique, it is essential to comprehend the role that carbs play in the diet.

The Function of Carbohydrates in the Body

Carbohydrates are essential for maintaining general health and well-being. They are the brain and muscles' preferred energy source, supporting both mental and physical activity. Carbohydrates help several body systems function well when taken in the right amounts. On the other hand, an imbalance in the consumption of carbohydrates can result in problems with weight and other health difficulties.

Different types of carbohydrates

There are two types of carbohydrates: simple and complex, each with unique properties. Simple carbs cause a sharp jump in blood sugar levels because they are rapidly absorbed and can be found in refined grains and sugary foods. Complex carbs, found in whole grains, fruits, and vegetables, on the other hand, take longer to digest and release energy gradually. Comprehending the distinctions between these two categories of carbohydrates is crucial in formulating a successful carb cycling scheme.

How Carbs Affect Blood Sugar Levels

The levels of blood sugar are directly impacted by the consumption of carbs. Simple carbs can cause blood sugar to rise and fall quickly, which can exacerbate sensations of hunger and exhaustion. Complex carbs, on the other hand, cause glucose to be released more gradually and steadily, resulting in stable energy levels. An important aspect of the carb-cycling diet is controlling how much of a negative effect carbs have on blood sugar to maximize energy use and general metabolic health.

CHAPTER ONE

The Carb Cycling Diet's Foundations

The Carb Cycling Diet is a nutritional strategy designed to maximize energy levels, encourage fat reduction, and improve overall performance by alternating the consumption of carbohydrates on different days or at particular times.

People who are looking for a flexible and long-lasting approach to control their weight and enhance their body composition have become more and more interested in this diet.

What Is Cycling On Carbs?

A dietary approach known as "carb cycling" aims to vary the quantity of carbs taken in over a week or within a specified period.

In contrast to conventional diets that recommend consuming macronutrients consistently throughout the day, carb cycling alternates between periods of higher and reduced carbohydrate intake. This variance frequently corresponds with a person's training regimen or degree of exercise.

How Cycling Carbs Operates

The main idea of carb cycling is to systematically time your consumption of carbohydrates to satisfy your body's energy needs. People may eat more carbs on days when they exercise more or physically exert themselves more to restore glycogen levels and supply the energy needed to operate.

In contrast, carbohydrate intake should be minimized on rest or lower-intensity training days to promote the body's use of fat reserves as an energy source.

Cycling on carbs makes use of the way that carbs affect insulin levels.

Increased insulin production from a higher carbohydrate diet can support the growth of muscles and the storage of glycogen.

Conversely, consuming less carbohydrates may increase fat burning because, when glycogen stores are depleted, the body switches to burning fat for energy.

Diverse Methods For Cycling Carbs

There are several ways to carb cycle, and people can select the one that best suits their interests, lifestyle, and fitness objectives.

One popular strategy is to alternate throughout the week between days with high, moderate, and low carbohydrate counts.

An alternative strategy is to time your carbohydrate consumption to correspond with particular training phases. For example, you may consume more carbs during a period of bulking or muscle gain and less during a phase of cutting or fat reduction.

Some people might choose a more haphazard strategy, modifying their daily activity levels and energy needs to determine how much carbohydrates they should consume.

This adaptability enables a customized approach to carb cycling that takes into account each person's particular requirements and preferences.

Apart from adjusting the amount of carbohydrates consumed, the Carb Cycling Diet frequently highlights the significance of upholding a well-rounded diet. Sufficient protein and good fats are essential for maintaining muscle mass, promoting fullness, and meeting general dietary requirements. Making nutrient-dense food choices and monitoring micronutrient intake is critical to a well-rounded and long-term approach to nutrition.

The Carb Cycling Diet is a dynamic and adaptable method of controlling carbohydrate consumption, enabling people to customize their diets to suit their specific needs and training schedules. As part of their overall fitness and wellness journey, those looking for a flexible and periodized nutritional strategy can find value in investigating the ideas of carb cycling, albeit it might not be appropriate for everyone.

CHAPTER TWO

Setting Goals For Your Carb Cycling

A dietary strategy called "carb cycling" is adjusting the amount of carbs consumed on a daily, weekly, or monthly basis. Before starting a carb cycling diet, it's important to have certain objectives.

Whether you want to lose weight, gain muscle, or improve your athletic performance, knowing what your goals are can help you customize the carb cycling strategy to suit your requirements.

Loss Of Weight

Losing weight is one of the main reasons people follow a carb-cycling diet. The goal of this strategy is to control the amount of carbohydrates consumed to maximize fat burning while maintaining lean muscle mass.

The body is urged to use fat reserves as fuel on low-carb days, which aids in weight loss. Glycogen stores are refilled on high-carb days, keeping the body from going into a state of deprivation that could impair metabolism and cause muscle loss.

Generally, low-carb and high-carb days are alternated while using carb cycling to lose weight.

Reduced calorie and carbohydrate consumption can be indicative of low-carb days, although enhanced energy and muscle glycogen repair is possible on high-carb days. It is thought that this cyclical pattern will improve metabolic flexibility and encourage long-term, sustainable weight loss.

Building Muscle

It is possible to modify carb cycling to promote goals other than weight loss, such as muscle growth. Increased carbohydrate consumption gives the body the fuel it needs to support hard training sessions and muscle repair.

For those who are doing strength training and other muscle-building exercises, this is very advantageous.

The focus is on refueling glycogen storage and supplying the energy required for strenuous exercise on high-carb days. This can improve gym performance and lead to more effective training sessions. Furthermore, consuming more carbohydrates these days encourages the release of insulin, a hormone essential for the synthesis of muscle protein. The preservation and increase of lean muscle mass are facilitated by this combination of factors.

Enhanced Athletic Capabilities

An important tactic for athletes trying to maximize their performance is carb cycling.

Athletes can carefully schedule high-carb days around demanding training sessions or contests thanks to the diversity in carbohydrate consumption. They can guarantee that glycogen stores are optimized in this way, offering an easily accessible energy source for high-intensity exercises.

A higher diet of carbohydrates can enhance endurance and minimize exhaustion during times of heightened physical effort, such as intense training sessions or competitive activities. In contrast, a decreased carbohydrate diet may be suitable to promote overall energy balance on rest or low-intensity days. This customized strategy for carbohydrate intake fits the unique requirements of an athlete's training and competition calendar to improve overall performance.

CHAPTER THREE

Forming A Plan For Carb Cycling

A nutritional approach called "carb cycling" entails changing your daily, weekly, or monthly carbohydrate consumption.

Optimizing performance, promoting fat reduction, and enhancing muscular growth are the objectives.

It's crucial to take into account elements like daily calorie intake, macro ratios, and a well-organized cycle schedule when developing a carb-cycling diet.

Finding Your Daily Calorie Need

Establishing your daily calorie intake is a fundamental step in creating a carb-cycling diet. This entails figuring out how many calories your body requires to stay at its current weight.

In this computation, variables like height, weight, gender, age, and degree of exercise are important. You can then modify your consumption depending on your fitness goals, such as weight reduction, maintenance, or muscle gain, once you've determined your baseline caloric demands.

Finding The Macro Ratios

Comprehending the appropriate ratio of macronutrients, which include proteins, carbohydrates, and fats, is crucial for an effective carb cycling regimen.

The way these macros are distributed can affect how much energy is available, how muscles are preserved, and how fat is used.

Carbohydrates give us energy, lipids help regulate hormones, and protein is essential for muscular growth and repair.

The precise macro ratios may change depending on workout intensity, metabolic rate, and personal preferences.

Creating A Cycling Timetable

Creating an organized riding plan is the key to successful carb cycling.

To accomplish certain goals, this entails deliberately switching between days with high and low carbohydrate content. Low-carb days are intended to encourage fat-burning and high-carb days are frequently planned around rigorous exercise sessions to support performance and aid in recuperation.

To find a balance, some people might incorporate a day with modest carbs. Cycling frequency and pattern can be tailored to an individual's response to varying carbohydrate levels, lifestyle, and fitness regimen.

You may maximize your body composition and performance by carefully planning a cycling routine that synchronizes your nutritional intake with your exercise demands.

Being adaptable is essential because it lets you make changes according to how your body reacts to the riding technique.

To follow through on the carb cycling diet and achieve long-term success, it is imperative to track progress and make appropriate adjustments.

The carb-cycling diet is a sophisticated strategy that calls for careful preparation and modification.

Every element is essential to reaching the intended fitness goals, from figuring out macro ratios and creating a cycling routine to computing daily calorie intake. A well-designed carb cycling plan can be a useful tool in your nutritional toolbox, regardless of your goals—weight loss, muscle gain, or improved athletic performance.

CHAPTER FOUR

Days Of High Carb:

Including high-carb days in the diet is an essential part of the Carb Cycling Diet. Compared to low-carb days, these days are defined by a higher intake of carbs. Incorporating high-carb days is intended to replenish glycogen stores, which may be exhausted during low-carb times.

It is thought that this replenishment of glycogen supports energy levels, improves performance during exercise, and wards off exhaustion.

Goal And Advantages:

The main goal of adding high-carb days to the Carb Cycling Diet is to provide the body with a brief boost in carbohydrate consumption to help it fulfill energy needs.

It is believed that this cyclical strategy prevents the metabolic adaption that long-term low-carb diets can cause. High-carb days are also thought to cause the release of insulin, a hormone that is essential for the synthesis of muscle protein and the transportation of nutrients.

Increased muscle mass is possible, improved recovery from exercise, and higher exercise performance are all advantages of high-carb days.

This method is frequently used by athletes and fitness enthusiasts to maximize their training schedule and achieve their fitness objectives.

Foods To Eat On High-Carb Days:

To get the most out of the Carb Cycling Diet, you must select the appropriate foods for your high-carb days.

Whole grains, sweet potatoes, oats, and brown rice are examples of complex carbs that are frequently advised.

These foods slow down the release of energy, which keeps blood sugar levels from rising and falling too quickly. Lean proteins and healthy fats can also contribute to the creation of a well-balanced meal that meets dietary requirements on all fronts.

An Example Of A High-Carb Day Menu:

A sample high-carb day meal plan must balance macronutrients to guarantee that the right amounts of fats, proteins, and carbohydrates are consumed.

A high-carb day could begin with a breakfast consisting of fruit and oatmeal accompanied by a protein source, like Greek yogurt or eggs.

 Quinoa salads, grilled chicken with sweet potatoes, and rice cakes with nut butter could be some of the day's snacks and dinners. It's critical to customize the meal plan to meet dietary needs and personal tastes while keeping the overarching goal of consuming more carbohydrates on these particular days.

With its focus on days with high and low carbs, the Carb Cycling Diet provides a versatile and dynamic approach to nutrition.

Many people use this method to support their general well-being and fitness goals, though the scientific evidence for its efficacy is still developing. Before making big adjustments to one's eating habits, it is advised to speak with a healthcare provider or a qualified dietician, as with any diet.

CHAPTER FIVE

Dead Carb Days

A key component of the Carb Cycling Diet is No Carb Days, which limit your intake of carbohydrates for a certain amount of time.

The idea behind this strategy is to cause a change in the body's metabolism so that fat reserves are used for energy rather than carbs.

A well-planned integration of No Carb Days into the overall dietary pattern may help people lose fat more effectively while maintaining muscular mass.

Goal And Advantages

To optimize fat burning, the main goal of adding No Carb Days to the Carb Cycling Diet is to change the body's metabolism. Insulin levels fall during carbohydrate restriction, causing the body to use fat reserves as a source of energy.

Over time, this may help with weight loss and better body composition. Furthermore, No Carb Days might aid people with specific medical disorders by lowering inflammation and regulating blood sugar levels.

Perfect Meals To Avoid Carbs

It's important to make the appropriate meal choices on No Carb Days to follow the guidelines of the Carb Cycling Diet and preserve nutritional balance.

These days, the main ingredients of meals are healthy fats, lean proteins, and non-starchy veggies. Low-carb veggies like leafy greens, broccoli, cauliflower, and spinach are great options, and lean protein sources like fish, poultry, and turkey offer the necessary amino acids. Nuts, avocados, and olive oil are good sources of healthy fats that promote overall well-being and satiety.

An Example Of A Low-Carb Day Menu

Making a tasty and well-balanced meal plan for Carb Days is crucial to following the Carb Cycling Diet. Breakfast on a regular day can consist of scrambled eggs with avocado and spinach, which provides healthy fats and protein.

 A tasty and low-carb lunch option is grilled chicken breast served with roasted broccoli on the side and a salad made with cucumbers, cherry tomatoes, and leafy greens.

A dish of cauliflower rice and baked fish with asparagus maybe dinner.

A handful of nuts or sliced cucumber with guacamole are examples of snacks that provide a variety of nutrients without being overly high in carbohydrates.

The Carb Cycling Diet's No Carb Days offer a calculated method for controlling carbohydrate intake, encouraging fat reduction, and maximizing metabolic efficiency. People can customize their diet to reflect their unique objectives and tastes by learning about the rationale, advantages, and best foods to eat on No Carb Days.

CHAPTER SIX

Fitness And Carb Cycling Combined

For best effects, carb cycling can be used with other workout modalities synergistically. This section examines the mutually beneficial relationship between exercise and carb cycling, highlighting the significance of matching dietary plans to particular training objectives.

Whether the goal is to increase muscle mass, reduce body fat, or improve athletic performance, smart carb cycling can be a useful addition to a variety of training programs.

Exercise For The Heart

This section describes the function of carb cycling for those who are adding cardiovascular exercise to their fitness routine to maximize energy levels and enhance endurance.

There are guidelines for modifying the amount of carbohydrates consumed according to the kind, level of intensity, and length of aerobic exercise, which provides a thorough method for supplying the body with fuel for aerobic activity.

Strength Development

Carb cycling can be very beneficial for strength training aficionados if they customize their carbohydrate intake to promote muscle growth and recovery.

This section explores the connection between strength training and carb cycling, including suggestions for days with high and low carbs to improve performance, encourage the synthesis of muscle protein, and speed up recovery.

When To Work Out Using Carb Cycling

The advantages of carb cycling can be increased by carefully coordinating your intake of carbohydrates with your exercise routine.

The significance of pre- and post-workout nutrition about carb cycling is explained in this section. Useful advice on modifying carbohydrate intake according to training session scheduling is offered to maximize energy use, encourage recovery, and successfully meet fitness objectives.

The Carb Cycling Diet presents itself as an adaptable and customized approach to nutrition, providing a sophisticated method of controlling carbohydrate consumption in line with personal requirements and athletic goals.

People can maximize the benefits of carb cycling for better health, performance, and general well-being by combining it with exercise and using an informed approach to meal planning.

Troubleshooting Typical Problems

Weight reduction Plateaus: With any diet, it's normal to encounter weight reduction plateaus. Reefed days, calorie intake, and macronutrient ratio modifications may be taken into consideration to help overcome this carb cycling difficulty.

Handling Cravings:

Cravings can be difficult to deal with, especially on low-carb days. To address this problem, choose satiating and nutrient-dense foods, drink plenty of water, and schedule deliberate refeed days to satiate cravings without impeding progress.

Modifying The Diet For Particular Situations

Athletes and Performance Objectives: To meet particular training requirements, athletes may need to customize their carb cycling regimen. Performance and recuperation can be maximized by modifying the ratios of macronutrients according to the duration and intensity of workouts.

Medical problems and Dietary limitations: Before starting the Carb Cycling Diet, anyone with medical problems or dietary limitations should speak with qualified dietitians or other healthcare providers.

To meet specific health issues and guarantee that nutritional demands are addressed, customization is essential.

A customizable and adaptable approach to eating, the Carb Cycling Diet can help achieve a range of fitness and health objectives. An effective and long-lasting carb cycling experience will come from comprehending the fundamentals, using the plan with consideration, and resolving obstacles.

CHAPTER SEVEN

Changing To A More Sustainable Way Of Eating

Long-term success with carb cycling requires a shift from a strict cycle to a more sustainable eating habit.

This entails striking a balance between your fitness and health objectives and your lifestyle and tastes.

Including Cycling On Carbs In Your Lifestyle

To successfully integrate carb cycling into your lifestyle, you need to be organized and reliable. Meal planning, monitoring your intake of macronutrients, and maintaining awareness of your energy usage may all be part of this. Long-term enjoyment and sustainability of carb cycling can be increased by modifying recipes and developing a varied meal plan.

Keeping An Eye On And Modifying Your Plan As Needed

It's critical to track your progress and adjust as needed as your body adjusts to carb cycling.

This could entail adjusting the duration of high- and low-carb cycles, adjusting the macronutrient ratios, or reevaluating your total caloric intake.

Consultations regularly with a dietitian or healthcare provider can yield insightful advice and direction for sustained success.

Long-Term Upkeep And Integration Of Lifestyle

The key to successful carb cycling over the long run is incorporating it into your entire way of life.

This entails considering carb cycling as a long-term dietary pattern rather than a quick diet.

The long-term benefits of carb cycling depend on finding a balance that supports your fitness objectives, enhances your health, and meets the demands of your everyday life.

Stories Of Success

Success stories from real life offer important insights into the viability and efficacy of the carb-cycling diet.

People who have used this strategy share their stories, illuminating the difficulties they encountered, the tactics that helped them, and the observable outcomes they were able to get.

For those who are thinking about including carb cycling into their nutritional plan or are already doing so, these success tales can be an inspiration.

Individuals' Actual Experiences with the Carb Cycling Diet

Testimonials & Stories Of Transformation

Testimonials and success stories provide an intimate look into the lives of those who have adopted the carb-cycling diet. These personal accounts offer a sophisticated perspective on the many effects that carb cycling can have on individuals.

These stories demonstrate the adaptability of carb cycling and its potential to positively influence several areas of an individual's health and well-being, from weight loss and improved body composition to enhanced sports performance.

To sum up, the carb cycling diet is a flexible nutritional strategy that can be tailored to each person's needs and tastes. Through deliberate switching between days with high and low carbs, people may be able to improve their energy, body composition, and general health. Even if testimonies and success stories highlight the beneficial experiences of certain followers, people must approach carb cycling carefully, taking into account their particular situation, and seeking medical advice when necessary.

Conclusion

The carb-cycling diet is a sophisticated nutritional strategy that can work well for people who want to maintain their muscle mass while losing fat. Participants in this dietary regimen may benefit from enhanced metabolic flexibility and optimal energy use by carefully adjusting their intake of carbohydrates.

This section offers a succinct summary of the main ideas covered in the carb cycling topic. Readers are reminded of the basic ideas, the science underlying the methodology, workable implementation techniques, and the possible advantages and difficulties of carb cycling.

Motivation For The Future Journey Of The Reader

Starting a new diet, like carb cycling, takes commitment and persistence. Readers will find encouragement in this last section, which will help them to stick to their fitness and health objectives. It promotes a positive outlook and highlights the significance of customization and gradual modifications for a successful carb cycling experience.